# WHY WAIT?

## A HOSPICE CALL TO LIFE

JOSEPH H. SCHLERETH

*Garrick Birth - 2-26th*
*Lrrie's Birth = 11-2nd*

**DORRANCE**
PUBLISHING CO
EST. 1920
PITTSBURGH, PENNSYLVANIA 15238

The contents of this work, including, but not limited to, the accuracy of events, people, and places depicted; opinions expressed; permission to use previously published materials included; and any advice given or actions advocated are solely the responsibility of the author, who assumes all liability for said work and indemnifies the publisher against any claims stemming from publication of the work.

All Rights Reserved
Copyright © 2019 by Joseph H. Schlereth

No part of this book may be reproduced or transmitted, downloaded, distributed, reverse engineered, or stored in or introduced into any information storage and retrieval system, in any form or by any means, including photocopying and recording, whether electronic or mechanical, now known or hereinafter invented without permission in writing from the publisher.

Dorrance Publishing Co
585 Alpha Drive
Pittsburgh, PA 15238
Visit our website at *www.dorrancebookstore.com*

ISBN: 978-1-4809-5706-0
eISBN 978-1-4809-5729-9

# Contents

Foreword - by Joe Schlereth . . . . . . . . . . . . . . . . . . . . . . . . . . v
Chapter 1: To Speak Freely . . . . . . . . . . . . . . . . . . . . . . . . 1
Chapter 2: The Coexistence of Faith and Fear . . . . . . . . . . . 7
Chapter 3: Peace and Acceptance . . . . . . . . . . . . . . . . . . . 13
Chapter 4: A Cheerful Heart Is Good Medicine . . . . . . . . 19
Chapter 5: What to Do with Pain . . . . . . . . . . . . . . . . . . . 25
Chapter 6: Unfinished Business . . . . . . . . . . . . . . . . . . . . 29
Chapter 7: Pride . . . . . . . . . . . . . . . . . . . . . . . . . . . . . . . . 33
Chapter 8: Love . . . . . . . . . . . . . . . . . . . . . . . . . . . . . . . . 37

# Foreword

This book is an eyewitness account of sorts of the scene of a most opportunistic event; one in which some of us will participate someday, while others will only see vicariously. The goal is to present an expansion of the experience known as "dying" to the reader. I'm defining dying in this context to be the time between when we know or are told we are dying and when physical death actually occurs.

Let me offer a converse illustration to more clearly explain. When I was young, and the subject of dying was discussed by adults, many of them would conclude the matter by saying, "I just want to be hit by a truck." Their goal was mainly focused on eliminating suffering. As I contemplate these discussions, I wish I could go back and expound. You see, they only seemed concerned about the physical dimension of dying. As a hospice nurse of sixteen years, I've never seen death involve only the physical aspect of anyone involved, whether it be a patient, caregiver, family member, or friend.

As we live our lives, most of us get so busy that we don't take the time to reflect on our whole selves. After all, the physical is often what the world measures. The internal person—our spiritual, psychological, and emotional being—sees limited or even optional duty. One of our goals in life should be to truly incorporate all of our facets so that none are optional.

Sadly, many of us require an epiphany for this to happen. The person hit by a truck has no time to re-evaluate. There's no time to look at our respective values or our spiritual awareness. Given the opportunity to do this, which individuals commonly experience through hospice, often results in changes in actions and attitudes. This part of life that I have called dying is one denied to the "hit-by-a-truck" victim. Neither person may have needed a motivation toward spiritual awakening, but then again, maybe both did.

An expansion of this look at dying should serve to enrich our lives. The stories and lessons patients and caregivers have shared with me throughout the following pages may be a purging to some and an affirmation to others. Whichever the case, the lessons are pure and very possibly overdue. Concepts like reconciliation, peace, hope, joy, respect, and love are seen as the virtues they truly are.

It's a great privilege to recount some of these stories and share them with you. For those of you who are healthy while reading this, don't wait for that truck to come or for bad news from your doctor. Instead, consider what you could do to enrich the world and your life now. To those who've had the experience of tragedy, read these stories knowing your sufferings are not in vain. The wisdom you've gained has been earned, and it will far outlast the pain.

A few months ago, our hospice team was caring for a lady named Geraldine. Her family brought me to a special place as poignantly as any family has. The metaphor of a play came to mind, and I call it "Common Need."

## Common Need

> They give me presence in their hour of grief as if
> ushering me to the front row of their tragedy.

The lines are few and unnecessary as the cast is pulled out of themselves toward an expanse of common need.

Then they dim the footlights and invite me on stage, and all of us serve in various supporting roles.

It is profoundly appropriate that, for this hour, there is no distinction of position or degree of importance, except for the one for whom the play was written.

The closing curtain will punctuate this void and restore the rest of us to our hierarchy.

As we leave the theater and go our separate ways, we will ever remember and know how this star gave the performance of a lifetime to meet this common need.

The common need of love.

My writing comes from my Christian worldview, but I would contend many of the principles cross faith lines, and the accounts are worth considering. It causes me to remember the rhetorical words of the Apostle Paul, "O death, where is thy sting? O grave, where is thy victory?" (1 Cor. 15:55). Too many times I have looked into the eyes of a dying one to not consider the whole person during this occasion of physical death.

I'm eternally grateful to all who have touched my life in so many ways and have helped me see the reality of faith by what it accomplishes in our lives.

## Chapter 1

## To Speak Freely

One of the things I want to mention early on is my previous life experience as a production worker in several different factories in my hometown of Pittsburgh, Pennsylvania. I would like to think history has added a bit of color to my perspective.

I spent twenty years "blue collar" before my now 14 years "white collar" as a nurse. In the factory environment, the difference between us hourly workers and the salaried folks was the percentage of time we spent saying what we didn't mean. The freedom to say what you meant was inversely proportional to the perceived importance of your job.

We never heard managers say things like, "This place is really messed up," even when it was.

These factories were pretty dusty places when I spent my time there in the 1970s, so it wasn't uncommon for us working folk to write our thoughts on any relatively flat surface. An often-used acronym at our home away from home was "TPS." TPS was a bond the hourly employees connected with for suffering through our similar struggles of life in our small corner of the world. We weren't trapped in a true caste system, but it made us feel less alone to share a common resentment for something. You see, our secret mantra of TPS—"This Place Sucks"—was usually said with a smile on our faces. It was abundantly clear the managers felt the same way, but they knew they couldn't speak as freely as us. Unbeknownst to me at the time was how liberating it is to simply say what you thought.

As I stepped into the nursing arena, the expectation changed. Without my agreement or foreknowledge, I was now considered a manager, and the five years I spent in nursing facilities molded my speech to the accepted protocol.

Then hospice came along, and I was given the opportunity and the permission by patients and their families to once again be "common." This knowledge was not automatically clear to me, but fostered gradually through growing relationships.

When I meet a family in my role as a hospice nurse, I take care to let them lead in topics of discussion so as to not be insensitive to their grief, unless it's essential to their care.

I never ever tell the first joke (but I do have a few if you're interested).

I find there's a process of dialogue that becomes freer as time passes. I don't just mean for me, as the outsider, but also between family members and friends. The new topics are often like the elephant in the room, and there's a process of determining what can be said when, and to whom. Some patients and families who've had open communication lines before an illness now see these topics as too big to wrap their minds around. It is, however, beneficial to relationships to be able to talk about important matters, especially when there's the real possibility that their earthly relationship will soon end.

Sometimes, the patient and family members are each thinking they're protecting the other by working out their grief independently, but nothing could be farther from the truth.

With rare exception, there will be regrets by those surviving if the ability to speak freely isn't achieved. If there's unfinished business, it needs to be addressed.

Hospice chaplains and social workers see this as the primary focus of their work with families. Once relational issues are resolved, the more peace can serve. Once the elephant in the room is gone, the act of dying becomes a joint effort in creatively finding new paths each person's living will take.

Let me be clear that I'm not advocating wanton honesty that bears no respect for the feelings of others. We've all met people who think they're virtuous because they say what they think; the ones who leave a wake of brokenness because they have no deference. I'm *not* talking about this malevolent freedom. I'm talking about constructive communication borne out of mutual love and respect.

Fred Rogers was quoted as saying,

> "It is only natural that we and our children find many things are hard to talk about, but anything human is mentionable, and anything mentionable can be manageable. The mentioning can be difficult, and the managing too, but both can be done if we are surrounded by love and trust."

There's a parallel I've noticed as I'd been given instruction by a hospice chaplain and friend regarding a Catholic sacrament.

Quite some years ago, Last Rites were performed by priests as a parishioner lied on his death bed. I thought until recently this was still the case, but I have found that many Catholics see this ritual as a great comfort also. What I have learned is that it is now called the Sacrament of the Sick. When I asked about the appropriateness for having this performed, I found that it is helpful to have it done when a person is diagnosed with a terminal illness. The sacrament then serves the purpose of awareness to the individual that God is present for them throughout the course of their disease. It need not be repeated once it is done, and it offers peace, hope, and comfort to the patient and the entire family.

Just as it makes perfect sense to call on God as early as possible, it is also helpful to the whole circle of friends and family to draw closer to each other as soon as possible.

As I draw this parallel, it's obvious to me that when a suffering family can speak freely of their feelings early on, more healing work gets done with relationships, fewer anxiety medications are needed, less outside therapy is required during bereavement, and quality of life is generally better. There are even times when a plateau or reversal of symptoms follows that can be fully enjoyed and/or attributed to this congruence of body and mind. Many testimonials of this are given in Bernie S. Siegel's book, "Love, Medicine, and Miracles."

As I walk the streets of my town these days, I occasionally see Robert, the son of an elderly gentleman I helped care for about four years ago. When I was seeing his father, John, I also met Patricia, the daughter of the patient. Patricia was a successful woman with many responsibilities. Robert was unemployed and by most accounts not very well qualified as a caregiver. Without hesitation, however, and to the amazement of Patricia, Robert stepped in and took full responsibility for the care of his father.

Bricklayers don't generally have a natural affinity for changing diapers—especially their fathers'—but nothing slowed Robert down. It was only two short weeks that Robert served in this capacity to his father, but here is what was gained:

- Robert used this time to express his love in word and deed toward his father.

- Patricia gained new respect for Robert, for setting aside his destructive tendencies.

- The dying father witnessed his children getting along and was given a great sense of peace.

- And I got to see it happen.

- John died in peace due to his children's honest response to a difficult situation.

I should add that Patricia didn't shrink back in telling Robert she didn't expect him to do this. Even John told Robert this. I now have a bond with Robert. You see, Robert saw me as his lifeline when he needed it most. My minor, supportive role was major in Robert's eyes.

When I look at the work families and friends do when they think life is at stake and see the positive effects it creates, I can't help wishing it were something that could be done sooner. I contend that there would be more healthy relationships if we practiced more of this congruence in love.

Congruence means merely being honest about who we are and what we think and feel. Countless times, our terms of endearment are saved for dramatic events, when they would mean so much more if we said them for no particular reason at all. You never know when a seemingly random display of love might build a bridge of heightened understanding. Too many of our friends have needs we know nothing about, a history of pain, or unfulfilled aspirations they tell no one. Being vulnerable is too risky for some. If this is true, what value are we to our friends?

Hospice has blessed me with the profound privilege of entering a family situation when they're vulnerable. That's why they open up. Their ability to trust is relative to their need to trust. At this point, if I were to violate that trust in any way, I would be worse than useless. For example, if someone saved you from drowning, they may be physically present in your life for only hours, yet you would consider them one of the five most important people in your life. That lifeline is sacred.

What is the lesson to be learned from this?

It is simple. Live your life in such a way as to provide a haven of trust to the people you know so that the vulnerability needed for deep relationships doesn't have to wait for the catastrophe of illness.

It may not be that the people I meet in my job as a hospice nurse decide they want to open up to everybody now that they've survived this valley. I just hope the relationships they had before will be better, or that their future relationships can be. In my job, ninety-nine percent of the time, there's a loved one that dies. This transition will be most difficult, but it's easier when shared.

Cultivate your friendships now. Establish their value. You will then be better prepared to form mutually beneficial and enriching friendships in the future.

## Chapter 2

# The Coexistence of Faith and Fear

When I go to Webster's to read the definition of "faith," it says, "Complete trust or confidence." If you're familiar with the Bible, you may be acquainted with Hebrews 11:1: "Now faith is being sure of what we hope for and certain of what we do not see." Both of these seem to be opposed to doubt.

When I consult Webster's for the definition of "fear," it reads, "Anxiety caused by real or possible danger, pain, etc."

Probably neither word needs to be defined for you, because we all have experience with both. They do coexist in all of us, and although not really opposites, faith suggests positive feelings, and fear usually serves the negative.

One of the facts about life is its mystery.

John Lennon was quoted as saying, "Life is what happens while you are making other plans."

Life is the ultimate common denominator, and the sheer living of it preoccupies us.

Death is so abstract, it is easier mislaid.

There are some great words in a song the Christian rock group, Petra, sang years ago, called "Grave Robber."

> "There's a step that we all take alone,
> An appointment we have with the great unknown.
> Like a vapor, this life is just waiting to pass—
> Like the flowers that fade, like the withering grass.
> But life seems so long, and death so complete—."

That last line quoted is true most of the time. The sad truth is, even when life is short, death is complete. The only difference is it must not be mislaid any longer.

As I watch people suffer with their disease, I see both faith and fear. They are inversely proportional.

The most obvious contrast I've witnessed was with a COPD patient named Albert.

Chronic Obstructive Pulmonary Disease (COPD) has differing acuity levels. In short, breathing becomes more difficult as time passes. So it was with Albert. He was actually on the hospice program twice. He hit a plateau for about two years, so we happily discharged him. After a while, however, he became more acutely ill again.

Albert was a man of strong faith and poor lungs. There are medicines that help with this shortness of breath, and Albert used them at will, but there's always a period of time for folks with COPD between when you feel the shortness of breath coming and when the medicine helps. Anxiety and fear accompany shortness of breath a hundred percent of the time. Even though Albert had a strong faith, breathing in life is simply not optional.

If you think and look back to the definitions above, you'll notice the apparent contradictions of the Hebrews definition. It can be said the definition itself has to be taken on faith. As I got to know Albert, the definition became clear to me. Faith was very real to him. It did include hope. He had an eternal perspective that led his whole family through the heavy trials of illness. His fear was temporal, but his faith was eternal. God took Albert home peacefully where both his body and spirit could be whole.

Fear also rears its ugly head in the spiritual realm. While physical fears are very real, such as shortness of breath or concern for how loved ones will fare after your death, the more pure inversion comes spiritually. This fear is very personal and makes me think of James.

I met James when his wife was in the final stages of cancer. She wasn't able to communicate, so dialogue just involved James and me.

James listed his religion as "Atheist." Since, as I mentioned earlier, I generally allow families to initiate topics, James and my discussions were limited to details of his wife's care— until the last day.

On that day, James knew his wife was close to death, and his thoughts began to look past that time.

James said, "I've never been a religious man, and I'm not about to start now."

I showed my best silent support, not quite knowing what to say next. (Never underestimate the value of simple presence!)

James then said, "She was everything to me. I don't know how I'm going to live without her."

This is the time, if it hasn't been broached yet, when I ask of a person's faith. Since James had already eliminated that option, I reminded him of his two children. I told him he should keep in touch with them in his wife's absence.

James nodded in affirmation, and his wife did die that day.

I lost touch with James for about a year and a half. Then one day I got a report that James was now the hospice patient.

I learned from James' daughters that he'd spent about nine months putting together a memorial for his wife—chronicling her life—to give to his children. Shortly after he finished, James developed cancer.

This time, I had about a month with James. His personality was still the same. He was still the analytical chemist. James was obviously tired though. He'd just turned ninety.

James began to reflect on his life and tried to measure its worth on some evasive scale. He'd done great work as a chemist, pioneering things of which I'd even heard about. He was proud of his two wonderful daughters. I'd let James linger on these topics because I assumed his "not about to start now" belief was still intact.

Much to my surprise, however, on one visit, James came out with, "What do you think happens to us when we die?"

I was caught quite off guard. After seeing his wife die and taking the time to reflect on his life, James had finally gotten to one of those questions we mislay!

I told James that I don't believe this is all there is and that I believe in life beyond physical death.

I have to leave the conclusion of James' story to God, because we were interrupted, and he quickly retreated to safety. His fear was still strong-arming his faith.

Before I had an opportunity to visit again, James was gone.

James is the reason I believe almost everyone gets to those questions. Faith and fear coexist in all of us on some level. Our humanity is never devoid of fear, and no matter how spiritual we are, our faith is never perfect.

Two things that seemed evident with James were that his earthly accomplishments were easily enumerated, but his divine purpose still needed to be answered. James' vocation and family were what he lived for here, and that's admirable, but the question of spiritual faith eluded him for ninety years.

I would suggest that the words of this great hymn sum up the Christian faith well and give a divine purpose that Albert found, while James did not.

## The Solid Rock

> My hope is built on nothing less than Jesus' blood and righteousness;
> I dare not trust the sweetest frame, but wholly lean on Jesus' name.
> On Christ the solid rock I stand; all other ground is sinking sand,
> All other ground is sinking sand.

The unknown nature of disease adds fear to the life of the people I meet in my job. Their faith needs to be up to the added strain of physical debility. The secret is practicing faith before illness comes, so that trust in God is learned through experience.

The proverbial "foxhole" prayer is heard by God just as well, but the difference comes as we look back. How many blessings were missed that God had prepared? How many times did we "walk through the valley of the shadow of death" alone (Psalm 23)? God desires a relationship with his creation while we're here. His spirit will take away your biggest fears if only you believe He can. We will struggle, but we will always have an advocate, a friend, and one who knows our sufferings. The rest of the verse to the Petra song mentioned earlier in this chapter says,

> "And the grave an impossible portion to cheat,
> But there's one who has been there and still lives to tell.
> There is one who has been through both Heaven and Hell,
> And the grave will come up empty handed that day.
> Jesus will come and steal us away."

If even James can ask the big questions, anyone can. It's just so much better when God is found able sooner.

## Chapter 3
# Peace and Acceptance

*(A chapter with my worldview)*

I hope I'm not sounding too philosophical with these chapter titles, but it's always been my desire to get to the point. Those abstracts mentioned in the foreword (peace, hope, joy) give life its flavor. We've been given a great gift to be able to be analytical and emotional, and the blending of these two God-given gifts should decrease the sense that either is a curse. It should instead allow for a sense of euphoria.

So it is with peace. The last emotion that comes to mind in the midst of trauma is peace. There is alarm, then grief. Whether anticipatory or present, grief can affect us totally.

C.S. Lewis does a great piece that is an "excerpt from a grief observed" to show its pervasiveness. There are five stages of grief: denial, bargaining, anger, depression, and acceptance. There's also evidence to show it's a healthy process, despite the apparent negatives. How much a family is able to function during a time of grief is relative to their acceptance.

I think it's irrational to think humans have the ability to accept suffering, and yet acceptance with a grudge is not acceptance at all.

This is where the water gets murky among my fellow fundamentalists. Should we accept a disease or circumstance? Shouldn't we expect healing as stated in James 5:14–15?

> "Is any one of you sick? He should call the elders of the church to pray over him and anoint him with oil in the name of the Lord. And the prayer offered in faith will make the sick person well; the Lord will raise him up. If he has sinned, he will be forgiven."

Isn't God in control? Doesn't God still heal? Why does He heal some and not others? Is healing contingent upon my faith?

These questions may be difficult to answer as I ponder them in my study while sipping tea, but when a forty-five year old man asks me these questions as I sit in his study—a room away from his dying wife—I'd better be able to offer more than a deer-in-the-headlights look.

How is comfort found? How is peace obtained so that acceptance is real?

I offer this answer now on paper, but I'm ever careful not to assume it's what that forty-five-year-old man wants to hear then. I offer it now and believe I can wrap my mind around it just enough to portray a sense of peace to him—peace instead of fear.

Although God is omnipotent, we have been given free will ever since the creation of the first man, Adam. The dominion over this Earth that was given to man (Genesis 1:28) was forfeited when sin entered the Earth (Genesis 3:15–19) through that free will. The Earth, man, woman, and the serpent were part of the curse, and death became the end result (Genesis 2:17 and 3:19).

In Luke 4:6, it's made clear who has dominion now on this Earth as the devil offers to return that charge to Jesus if He will only bow down and worship him. Jesus refuses most strongly.

The devil's goal is stated clearly in I Peter 5:8 where Peter says, "Be sober, be vigilant, because your adversary, the devil, like a roaring lion walks about, seeking whom he may devour."

God does not cause drought or flood or fire or murder or adultery. God's original design was not what we see in the world today. All of us, as descendants of Adam, suffer and die because of this separation from God. Although He hates sin and must separate Himself from us because of his holiness, He is also a God of love and has provided a way for us to return to Him.

So the best way for me to accept suffering and death is to assign its origin to whom it belongs—the devil. I know that it's temporary (Revelation 21:4) if we accept John 3:16, "For God so loved the world that He gave his only begotten Son, that whoever believes in Him should not perish, but have everlasting life." I live life with the peace that comes only from the Creator.

Remember when I said I've never seen death be only physical for those around it, and in the Foreword, I quoted I Corinthians 15:55? It's because of the reality of everlasting life. The verse again says, "Where, Oh death, is your victory? Where, O death, is your sting?"

Acceptance and peace are possible through a trust in God that this is not all there is. There was a glow on the face of Stephen when he was being martyred because he could see God's glory (Acts 7:54–60). Whatever this world has to offer temporarily is of little significance compared to what God offers permanently.

About three years ago, I was helping a family take care of their elderly father who had this peace in the midst of "dying." The family had taken a picture of him smiling in his hospital bed, arms behind his head, smoking a cigar. This man knew his God through a personal relationship with Jesus Christ. He practiced his faith daily so that he had a heavenly perspective on his life. His grief was manageable for him and his family, because his God was real. Though not within his control, his time of departure was seen with the hope of one finally going home.

His legacy was multiplied, because he found God's peace early in life. The picture showed a man looking through the eye of the camera at something much grander.

In case you see the man in that picture as one old enough to be ready to die, I want to add one more family's story here.

Jeff was only forty-four years old. He also had cancer. Jeff was the pastor of one of our local churches. He had three young children, aged four through twelve, and a beautiful wife. Jeff had a growing ministry with a positive effect on many, yet he is now gone from us.

In the five months I visited with Jeff and his family, they gave more to me than I did to them. I never heard, "Why me?" or "Why us?" What I saw was strength and courage and a sure trust in their God.

As diligent as they were in their ministry to others here on Earth, they had high hopes for a brighter day. Jeff even chose the sermon topic for the elder who would preside at his funeral service. It was from 2 Timothy:4, where Paul tells Timothy his departure is at hand. Jeff told the elder, "Don't you dare say I have died. I have only departed."

These two men and their families, as well as many others, taught me what peace and acceptance really are. They're mutually inclusive. Both families, and countless others (me included), were blessed because they sought and found their God early in life.

I would like to share one of my poems here. This poem is a tribute to a woman I met in 1996. She was the victim of a stroke. This lady helped me focus on what it really means to be whole, and where not to look for it.

## A Gift to Bring

The fragile life within our bodies make us all the same;
The way we live does fool us, though; we think we know our frame.
So on we plan for life's delights, while working when we must;

# Why Wait?

We handle things so well ourselves, that in ourselves we trust.
It is no crime, I will submit, to think that it is so.
But then the fate we have ignored grabs the life we know,
We lose control and ask, "Why me?" but to whom do we plead?
If someone's there to answer us, will they not meet the need?
The one who really knows us best looks more at each one's soul,
And uses that above all else to gauge who's really whole.

Well, I know such a lady now, whose body lies at rest;
She cannot talk, or move herself, to do what she likes best.
She can't say, "Leave," if silence is her simple need today;
The limits forced upon her heart bring untold pain her way.
We care for her and think we do a somewhat righteous thing,
But who helps whom in all the rush? Who has the gift to bring?
Well, I submit again, and say this lady helps us too;
Her eyes can let us see our soul more clearly than we do.
There's no pretense, no judgment seen, just openness I see;
She gives more than I ever will by helping me see me.

So when we care for you, my dear, remember what I said;
The deepest needs we have, you meet, just lying in that bed.

## Chapter 4
# A Cheerful Heart Is Good Medicine

This chapter will be devoted to a handful of humorous stories from hospice visits. The soberness of the whole situation adds to the effect, since, under normal circumstances, some of these tales would not be very funny.

As health care providers, at times we fall into the M*A*S*H mentality of finding humor in suffering, but these are instances where the patient or family surprises us.

The title for this chapter comes from Proverbs 17:22, which reads, "A cheerful heart is good medicine, but a crushed spirit dries up the bones." Laughter is a universal balm that has a way of connecting some of those facets within us. It has been proven to be just as the Proverb says.

### Mistaken Identity

One of my co-workers is a thirty-year-old nurse with a rather dry sense of humor. As she entered the home of her next visit one day, a dog ran in with her. It was the first time she'd visited this family, which consisted of the patient and her sister, both in their seventies. They made it through the initial introductions when Ellen noticed they seemed a bit pensive. It's not uncommon to see these emotions in families, since this is a stressful and emotional time. The ladies made their way up to the living room to sit and review the medicines and symptoms, and the dog jumped up on the couch with them.

There can be any number of underlying problems that are sorted out as time goes by. A few routine questions were answered by the sisters, when it seemed they really had something they had to ask.

"Excuse me," the one said, "but do you always bring your dog on your visits?"

Ellen responded in a puzzled tone, "Isn't that your dog?"

"No!" the exclaimed in unison, and the poor dog was escorted to the door. The rest of the visit was much more relaxed for everyone.

## The Hospice Flag

Many of our hospice families want us to keep in touch after the death of their loved ones, but this becomes impossible as time passes. As much as we like those we meet, the nature of the business (or perhaps I should say, life's "busy-ness") typically prohibits this.

I was seeing an elderly woman who remained quite stable for ninety percent of our visits, and yet I spent a lot of time there engaging with her husband. He was rarely able to get out, and he valued my visit more than most caregivers. Jim was a retired tugboat captain and shared many marvelous stories. He reminded me of a cross between Grandpa (from *The Real McCoys*) and Red Skeleton. Jim slyly introduced me to Limburger cheese, which I now know I don't like! He was creative and resourceful and even had a closed circuit TV set up so he could eat in the kitchen while watching his wife in the bedroom.

A key member of any hospice team is the nurse's aide. If the family desires this help, the aide also visits regularly. We were all quite impressed when the particular nurse's aide caring for Jim's wife showed up at the office one day with a "hospice flag" that Jim had sent back with her.

This special hospice flag was made from two blue disposable incontinence pads and decorated with black permanent markers. It seemed quite symbolic to us that Jim would use the one supply that would be easiest to deface as a way to honor us. Jim didn't mind that we laughed. He laughed too.

That flag hung in our office for a year, and it served as a constant reminder of Jim and his amazing ability to find some joy during his struggles.

### The Fingernail

Pete was short of breath from the day I met him. Everything Pete did was to conserve effort. To move, to eat, to bathe, and even to talk, caused shortness of breath. He usually had complaints, and I didn't mind hearing them, because his world had become so small and so difficult.

Even the thought of a haircut was ominous for Pete, because it would mean sitting in a hard-backed chair for fifteen minutes on the other side of the room. The barber was open to doing a house call, but the thought of it would make Pete nervous. His anxiety would even have him sending his wife down their alley in the winter to see if I was coming if I was five minutes late and hadn't called.

With this being the situation, it would've been easier to see Pete as an older man, wasting away, one who'd already lost his zest for life. He wasn't ready for the journey, though. As you can imagine, this was one of the last places I expected a laugh.

One day when I arrived, Pete proceeded to tell me his woe for the day. Absent-mindedly, while trimming his fingernails, he'd inadvertently trimmed his favorite nail. I asked Pete what the big deal was, and he said, "Sh—! Now I—*pant, pant*—can't pick my nose—*pant, pant*—and that is how I—*pant, pant*—keep all of the dry crap out of it—*pant, pant*—that collects from the oxygen! Sh—!"

You'd have thought someone had just shot Pete's best hunting dog. I tried to feel his pain, but the most I could achieve was an expression of mild disappointment, with a grin of course. He took no offense, because he knew I really did care.

### The Hamburger that Wasn't

Those in my age bracket don't know what it's like to be without fast food. McDonald's was around when I was born. So it was with Lawrence and his wife Sherry.

Cirrhosis of the liver had caused Lawrence to lose weight everywhere but his stomach. While he waited on a transplant list, Lawrence was weakened to the point of being bedbound. Still, Lawrence had more great stories than most to tell.

Lawrence spared no vulgarity, even in front of his wife, to the point of often embarrassing me for her sake. He would always grin as though he was doing it for the sole purpose of her red face.

Sherry didn't drive, and she worked the 3–11 p.m. shift, so she was always there when I visited.

Lawrence had many ways to keep himself occupied while in bed, and one of the most unique was his pellet gun. He had his family rig up a target in the next room, and he could practice at a range of about twenty feet.

I'd been visiting Lawrence for about three months when I arrived one day to find Sherry not there. Lawrence told me she had someone take her to a doctor appointment and would be back shortly.

Now, you can't see from the front door to the living room where we were in the house that day, so when Sherry returned home at about 10:30 a.m., she didn't realize I was there.

Sherry came grumbling in shouting, "Those #@$&* !$@&ers wouldn't make you a hamburger!"

When she came around the corner and saw me, Sherry's mouth dropped open. I looked at Lawrence; then I looked at Sherry. I grinned, watching the color drain from embarrassed Sherry's rosy cheeks while she tried in vain to retrieve the words.

Without skipping a beat, Lawrence spoke up. "We were just talking about your filthy mouth. Weren't we, Joe?"

We both laughed out loud, and it took Sherry at least four more visits to relax around me. I witnessed a new dimension to their relationship that day when I realized it was actually two-sided!

## Hospice Weekly

This next story is not really a job, but a picture. I've kept it on my desk as a reminder of a very special gentleman. It's the smiling man with the cigar I mentioned earlier.

John's world, much like Lawrence's, had also shrunk to one room as his weakness and wounds progressed. John was ready to die, and yet was still so full of life.

John had his family hang this particular picture on their refrigerator. He gave me instructions to tell no one about it, for fear he would be taken off hospice care since he looked so good.

I can't help but smile when I look at the picture now—three years after his death. He died on hospice in that bed he's pictured in, but not before he had the opportunity to give me my "lucky t-shirt"—a shirt he offered me because it became too small for him. You see, John's shirt was what I was wearing when I bowled the best series of my life the following week (298– 255–190 for a 743 series!!!).

It was John's heart, however, that was so enriching, since he rose above the earthly limits given to him to let his spirit soar. Peace and acceptance were evident in the picture, just like they were evident in John's life.

## Chapter 5
# What to Do with Pain

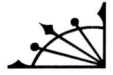 You may recall a previous chapter of this book that had a phrase in the introduction regarding grief:

"I think it's irrational to think humans have the ability to accept suffering."

On an even higher plane, in my opinion, is the thought of accepting pain. (And, of course, I'm speaking of willing acceptance again.)

When I was in the midst of writing this book, I was scheduled to have rotator cuff surgery to repair a large tear in my left shoulder. I'd injured it falling in my yard. Sharp pain accompanied certain movements of my arm, and I quickly learned what I couldn't do before the surgery. As I thought of the recovery time after surgery, I had visions of seeing this break from work as a great opportunity to write.

Wow, was I wrong! The pain after the surgery was pervasive mentally and physically, and the last thing I could do was put thoughts together.

My only consistent thoughts revolved around the clock, my pain, and being certain I wouldn't run out of pain medicine.

It wasn't that I wasn't told there would be pain. It wasn't that I didn't know what to do if I had pain. After all, I'm a hospice nurse! It was just that I'd never personally experienced this level of pain.

The nagging thoughts I recall as I survived each day of pain were those of considering what people do who face no end to this kind of pain? At least I had an expectation of future relief. Libraries could be filled with advice relative to pain management, so I won't spew any excessive blather. Instead, I'll give a brief outline of what I've seen tried through the use of one particularly instructive example and tell you most assuredly that I have a new awareness of pain's authority.

Pain is the body's way of telling us there's something wrong. With the people I see, the reason for the pain has been diagnosed. Hospice has palliation as its primary focus. Pain is present in most, and is generally accompanied by nausea, constipation, and anxiety.

Harold Steen had been working with his doctor for two years and had taken a big step by the time we met. Harold had an interthecal pump, an indwelling apparatus surgically placed to deliver pain medicine directly into his spine. It was the only way he could get relief. This basically blocked all sensation to his legs, and therefore he was unable to get out of bed.

Harold and his wife were two of the most pleasant folks our hospice team had the pleasure of serving. As you might imagine, the intervention of this pump brought with it new challenges for caretaking, but it was the lesser evil of the options Harold had.

Now, you may be wondering what connection there is between this drastic intervention to manage pain and willing acceptance. Let me tell you, they have everything in common.

I have no great story of healing from Harold, and I have covered my worldview quite sufficiently now, so I will provide some advice at this point.

## Why Wait?

The same God who created you gave the intelligence to some to create and use pain medicine. If you have pain, seek treatment. No one will fault you for managing your pain with prescribed medication, and I doubt anyone will give you a medal for withstanding unnecessary pain. If your doctor doesn't seem sensitive to your issues, get a second opinion. If your doctor has ever been in chronic pain, I doubt you will need a second opinion.

There are many misconceptions regarding pain medicine use. Your doctor, as well as your pharmacist, can dispel these myths. The only distinction I would make is the difference between acute and chronic pain. Both have their own treatment modalities, but both are manageable.

Chronic pain can be related to a terminal illness, or not, just as can acute pain. My only reason for adding in this afterthought chapter is because of my recent issues with pain. I see now how negligent it would have been for me to not mention pain.

If you have fears for a loved one, or for your own future in this area, I want you to be assured that pain can be managed, if not eliminated, with the appropriate attention. If you are the one in pain, it's very beneficial to have things in place so that someone can be your legal advocate if you cannot speak for yourself. Just as I spoke previously about performing the sacrament of the sick early in a diagnosis, so it should be with pain management.

After my recent episode with my shoulder, which is now improving with therapy, I can think of no greater comfort for my psyche than the management of physical pain. This may not be the longest or most profound or most pleasant of chapters, but if it's the only one you read, it's worth the price of admission.

I've had numerous families say, "I just don't want them to suffer."

How the grief is multiplied if pain is present. As much as the presence of pain pervades the one having it, it also interferes with the grieving process for those around the patient.

I hope I've made myself clear on what to do with pain, but as I close this subject, I must add that medicine isn't the only intervention, and if there's no terminal diagnosis, it's more of an adjunct therapy. From therapeutic touch to massage to music to laughter to surgery to meditation, and on and on—nobody needs to suffer needlessly. Seek help. Acceptance of pain intervention is the first step to accepting pain.

I wrote another poem a few years ago for those who suffer a different and sometimes silent pain. It's written in third person, as if from the Alzheimer's resident in a nursing home.

We cannot feel or understand their pain, but we should try to see them as God does and let Him use us in the encounter. Sometimes our presence is the best relief to the pain of another.

Each floor is a locked unit, where you must know the code of the keypad to leave.

## The Keypad

They give the wings names like "Bowman" or "Sheffield,"
As if it's an honor to guarantor such a place.
They paint the walls, tile the floor, and play their songs of choice,
And think their efforts prove their grace.
The valentines pasted on the doors, the flags, the trimmed tree
Are holidays devoid for me, lost in this keypad space.
The noises I hear are machines or people, but I can't tell from here
Since I'm just a wet diaper between meal trays.
Why don't they see the man in me unless they tear my skin?
It must be hard to see a soul through eyes that only gaze.
I don't know how I got here, because there is no way in or out.
My prison shrinks until I sleep all my fears away.
My only hope is somewhere there's a God who knows the code;
Then He'll walk in and rescue me from who I am today.

## Chapter 6
# Unfinished Business

I wrote a poem a few years ago called, "Life and Death." I wrote it prior to my hospice days. Its theme was that we should live in such a way that we're remembered for the good things, and that our death should be minimized. The fact is, death is usually a calm time, and most people do just "slip away." There's a country song that came out recently that has the theme of living like you were dying, by Tim McGraw. It is the idea of making every day count. Even my original title for this chapter was going to be "Live Memorably, Die at Peace."

I would like, however, to deal not so much with specifics here, but with a general principle. Matthew 5:13–16 speaks of how we're to be the salt of the Earth and light to the world. This implies that all of our actions must be taken with others in mind. No one lives alone. Even if you know someone who lives alone now, they didn't start out that way, and they won't end up that way. Even at the most basic level, we have to interact with someone. Where do we buy food or clothing? What's the exchange that puts the money in our hand? I don't think there will be much of an argument—we interact.

Of all the people I've met in my work, I've come to learn that the number of lives a dying one has touched is directly proportional to their willingness to be human. A bigger rock causes a larger ripple in the lake. (That is, of course, only if one throws oneself into the water.)

So it is with unfinished business. There can be many reasons for it—as many reasons as there are people we know. The happy person is the one who finds a way to be about their business—that is, always jumping in the water.

There's a tendency in our busy lives to ignore problems, to have to have our way on an issue, to disagree for some higher purpose, and then live this way for so long we forget how it started, or even that there was a start. I've known this to be true in my own life, so allow me to clarify.

As a line in the poem, "Life and Death," says, "each has worth in life." The things that diminish our lives, and those around us, are usually bitterness, pride, or fear.

For me, it was bitterness. My bitterness was due to an unforgiving spirit. That was a big unfinished business for me. There have been lesser ones through the years, but the wake-up call God gave me on that big one made me more aware of the little ones. There was more healing in that instance in my heart toward that person than I'd ever experienced, even though it wasn't mutual; and interestingly, I was then free to be more to other people in my life who had no connection to what caused that bitterness.

Some of the old spaghetti westerns used to use a line like, "Say your prayers, Mister," and this was the gun wielder's way of saying, "Get right with God, because you're about to meet him." This scenario isn't far from the "hit-by-a-truck" scenario. Even if you could fix it all right then, how much less would its value be than if you'd said your prayers every night?

I recently worked with a husband and dying wife who had everything in order—as they saw it. Early on, as we broached the question of dying. His reply was, "I told Jane she could go to sleep at night, because I would be watching. When I see the angel coming for her, I'll take his hand and put it in hers, and usher them away to Heaven. She has nothing to worry about."

Then Bernie would turn to Jane and say, "Isn't that right, Honey?" And Jane would not in affirmation.

Their children had visited a couple weeks ahead of her death, and Jane felt there was no unfinished business left.

The night of her departure, Bernie was there as he promised, and Jane passed peacefully.

We have so little time here, and so much of it is wasted. This couple enriched my heart forever. There was no bitterness, pride, or fear.

The Bible talks about faith, hope, and love. Only love crossed over with Jane. It was the bridge. Faith and hope were part of her life here, but they're completed and realized in heaven.

Make a difference in the day-to-day grind. Reflect the worth God sees in you. Let the collection of souls that gather around you have a long list with many years of stories about what you meant to them. Start with your family (as God first calls us to), and then ripple out like the rock in the pond.

## Chapter 7

# Pride

As I was taking a hiatus from these writings for another project, a thought came to mind with regard to our ill-timing of things. This is a tricky subject, because what determines the extent to which we relinquish our stubbornness has a lot to do with personality, not illness. Some of us easily cooperate with those close to us, even while healthy, understanding that our identity is based more on beliefs than who performs a certain household task.

I'm speaking to the person with illness now.

When I was in nursing school, as a matter of recognizing the profession as a discipline, we had numerous "nursing diagnoses." Whereas a medical diagnosis might be a fractured arm, a related nursing diagnosis for this would be "alteration in activities of daily living." This addresses the fact that there are activities we do that will be altered, and it is the nurse's job to educate about this.

Bear with me a little longer on this.

I might ask the victim, "Are you right- or left-handed," or "Do you live alone," or "What do you do for a living?" I would then know what goals to set, what interventions were needed, and what outcomes to expect.

Back to the illness.

With long-term illnesses, one such diagnosis is "role reversal." Role reversal can be difficult to overcome for those who are suddenly forced into the position of being dependent on someone who was previously dependent on them. Whether a sick woman who cannot concede the laundry to her husband or the sick man who cannot relinquish driving his car. Whether a grandchild now baking for grandma or grandpa, taking a job to help his daughter-in-law support his dying son—.

The touchy thing about role reversal is knowing that independence is healthy.

When do these changes happen? Who initiates them? What about the person who has always been happy to be waited on? What about safety?

Most times the doctor will tell you about the big things, like driving while on pain medication, or when to stop working. These are difficult to accept, so love and care must be the mode of operation when any changes are needed. A prerequisite of love and trust allows the transition. The presence of pride, however, often gets in the way, and can prove counterproductive.

To answer when these changes take place and who initiates them, it should be, "only when necessary," and "by you (the ill person)."

Notice I said "should be."

Unfortunately, it's been my experience that pride is the biggest hindrance.

Someone once gave me a pin that read, "If I don't do it, it doesn't get done." That's MY problem. I'm too sure of myself and don't like to be waited on.

When I had my surgery, I found myself raking leaves with one arm in a sling rather than asking my neighbor to help. He would have been glad to, and I could have very easily injured myself again—but I was too proud. (I'm working on that!)

I'll skip over the easily dependent person, because this chapter doesn't address them—they don't need it, and I'll move on to safety and the ramifications of doing unsafe things.

One of my patients, Tom, wouldn't give up his car key—until he wrecked. Fortunately, nobody was hurt.

Steven insisted on living alone—until he laid on the living room floor for six hours. He recovered, and then let his daughter move in.

William insisted on taking the stairs to shower—until he fell. Unfortunately, his wounds were fatal.

The point is that there are always choices. Maybe they're not pleasant ones, but they're still choices. Whatever the reason for resisting "role reversal" or any change, you must keep in mind the "cost." It's better to compromise to promote peace of mind than to have regrets.

One of the primary duties of our hospice team is to guide individuals through this process. We seek resources and promote communication.

One of the most difficult and challenging situations is the insidious disease of dementia.

As a caregiver, even in the most secure of settings—the home or a facility—safety is not a guarantee when dealing with an individual afflicted with dementia. Many unsafe situations can be managed, but falls may still be likely. Knobs can be removed from the stove, locks placed on doors, matches hidden, floors carpeted, even hot water tanks turned down, but you cannot be completely attentive twenty-four hours a day.

Everyone who is very ill gets weak, and it's the duty of caregivers, facility, staff, or professionals to provide as much safety to the mentally challenged as possible. The period of time someone is unsafe will last until they're too weak to get out of bed. This could be a period of a few days or it could be weeks. As a caregiver, you cannot beat yourself up if a loved one is injured. Have them treated as necessary, and continue on.

Excluding the mentally challenged from this issue of pride, here's how the "Why Wait" title applies here. In a true expression of love, relinquish your independence at such a time that your loved ones can offer optimum care. Then nobody will feel imposition, and those unnecessary emotions can be set aside, allowing for a fuller life experience until physical death.

## Chapter 8

# Love

Although I've been direct in my comments so far as they relate to my worldview, I'd like to address some of love's expressions first before the definition.

If I were to ask you to "define love," you may respond a thousand different ways. One way might be to say love is an action, and it's safe to say that definition is widely accepted. Anyone who's at least ten years past puberty will at least agree it's more than a feeling.

You might tell me how you've seen love expressed between a husband and wife, a parent and child, or life-long friends.

I believe love is a decision, and how it's expressed is usually how it's defined. But this really doesn't do love justice.

While this book talks rightfully so about feelings, we must remember feelings are given by God to serve us, not vice versa.

The world is the way it is today because of humans serving their feelings. Many emotions surface as we suffer through the trials of life, especially when the trial has the gravity of impending physical death. The only way to keep our balance is to have a decided base where truth is the buoy.

We examined fear when we compared it to the faith in our lives. Now we must look at love.

The song "Seasons of Love" from the popular musical "Rent" asks the question of how we measure a year in the life of someone. It asks, "In daylight, in sunsets, in midnights, in cups of coffee? In inches, and miles, and laughter, and strife? How do you measure a year in a life?" It finally sums up by asking, "How about love?"

This song evokes great mental pictures of how the daily, moment-by-moment events in life are what create the tapestry. Shouldn't we? Why couldn't we—measure it in love?

Romans 5:8 says, "But God demonstrates his own love for us in this: While we were still sinners, Christ died for us." John 3:16 is an elaboration of this same idea.

A short portion of 1 John:4 also says it beautifully in Verses 7–8: "Dear Friends, let us love one another, for love comes from God. Everyone who loves has been born of God and knows God. Whoever does not love does not know God, because God is love." There is the definition!

If God is love, then love = God. How did He express that love? By desiring a relationship with us through His Son, Jesus Christ. And how was that accomplished? By Jesus dying on the cross for our sins. The greatest news in the world is that we can know this love by getting to know God through Jesus Christ.

We spend most of our lives trying to self-empower with knowledge, trying to advance our positions by our own measurements, and doing so at such a pace that we think we're outrunning our fears of inadequacy and the pain of purposelessness. All we're really doing when left to ourselves is rearranging the chairs on a ship that's going down. The lifeline has been offered, and grabbing it will give you a focus through God's lens.

Yes, this is all by faith. No, you don't have to believe it.

My goal with all of the words in this book is to tell you what's worked for me. All of the people who work with me as we attend to those in need don't profess the same faith as me. It's not my job or duty to proselytize. It's not my goal to assert self, whether on the job or not. In fact, any attempt toward these things would be counter-productive.

My mission is to be an ambassador. It's to attend when there's nothing else that can be done. It's to seek relationships out of a necessity to meet common needs. It's to love out of excess. It's to give what has been given to me, to understand the value God places on every living soul, and to treat them accordingly.

If my faith had not convinced me of the urgency of these things, my profession would have. It's been a gift from God to have both!

The reading of this book won't serve the purpose of "how to do hospice," or "how to grieve," or even "how to live," but I hope it nudges you to introspection.

We all need to love, to be loved, and to have purpose. Don't spend one more day warming your hands on the fires of uncertainty. Set aside the fears of life, whatever yours are, because they will yield a lesser life for you and your loved ones.

One day my faith and hope will be proven, and then only love will remain. Tomorrow is not promised here on this Earth, so begin the pilgrimage today. Get to know "Love," and feel what it means to be blessed and to bless. You'll be exchanging masters. How much better to serve the one who made you and loves you than to serve yourself.

Oswald Chambers said, "Determinedly take no one seriously but God, and the first person you find you have to leave severely alone as being the greatest fraud you have known is yourself."

Physical death is but a step, and my prayer would be that the living of your life here would be full, no matter the length. I hope I have challenged you to examine the coexistence and codependence of death and life in order to both accept death and to truly live.

The words of Kahlil Gibran in "The Prophet" both express and transcend the Christian perspective on this matter:

And he said:
You would know the secret of death.
But how shall you find it unless you seek it in the heart of life?
The owl whose night-bound eyes are blind unto the day cannot unveil
The mystery of light.
If you would indeed behold the spirit of death, open your heart wide
Unto the body of life.
For life and death are one, even as the river and sea are one.

In the depth of your hopes and desires lies your silent knowledge of
The beyond;
And like seeds dreaming beneath the snow
Your heart dreams of spring.
Trust the dreams, for in them is hidden the gate to eternity.
Your fear of death is but the trembling of the shepherd when he
Stands before the king whose hand is to be laid upon him in his
Honour.
Is the shepherd not joyful beneath his trembling, that he shall wear
The mark of the king?
Yet is he not more mindful of his trembling?

For what is it to die but to stand naked
In the wind and to melt into the sun?
And what is it to cease breathing, but to free the breath from its
Restless tides,
That it may rise and expand and see God unencumbered?

Only when you drink from the river of silence shall you indeed sing.
And when you have reached the mountain-top, then you shall begin
To climb.
And when the earth shall claim your limbs, then shall you truly dance.
-*The Prophet, Kahlil Gibran*